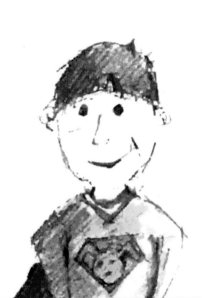

What is Cancer?
A Book for Kids

Carolina Schmidt

Illustrated by Bruno Calmon

Text: Carolina Schmidt

Illustration: Bruno Calmon

Diagramming: Carolina Schmidt

Cover: Carolina Schmidt, illustration by Bruno Calmon

Cataloguing-in-Publication Data (CIP)

Schmidt, Carolina, 1988.
   What is Cancer? A Book for Kids / Carolina Schmidt;
Illustration by Bruno Calmon. - Curitiba: Carolina Schmidt, 2015.

ISBN-13: 978-1522746737
ISBN-10: 1522746730

   1. Children's Literature.
I. Title II. Cancer III Schmidt, Carolina IV Calmon, Bruno.

1st edition revised and updated, 3rd update, 2018.

Most of us, kids, have contact with someone who has cancer: a relative or a friend; many children also have this disease.

If at any moment some adults were talking about cancer and noticed that we overheard them, they would start to whisper amongst themselves. They think that kids don't understand anything. In fact, adults are the ones who don't really understand.

The adults need hours and hours talking about cancer and asking other adults questions all of the time. Often, adults who are asked the questions know less than the ones who asked them.

Kids can understand these things. But many times, they don't know about them because they only hear the word "cancer" amid whispers, and nobody explains it.

What is this disease? Why do only adults talk about it? Why don't they tell me anything about it?

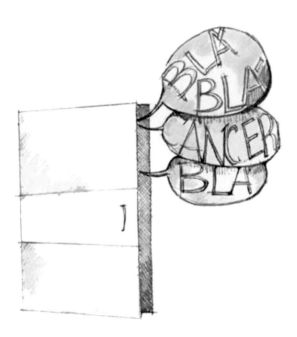

One day, I found out all these answers. I wasn't feeling well, so my parents took me to the hospital, where I got better. There, I heard adults whispering. Among the whispers, I heard the word "cancer".

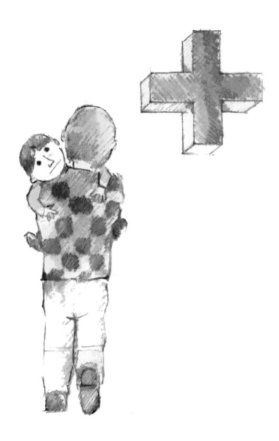

The word "cancer" echoed inside my head, because no one explained to me what it meant. I asked, and they told me that I should rest.

But what kid needs to rest when they just woke up?

Kids want to play, not sleep. I quickly got a notebook and a pencil. While my mother was sleeping, I snuck out of the hospital room. I went for a walk in the hospital.

I met a nurse in the hallway, and I tried to ask her everything about cancer, but I got no answers. She took me back to my room. I snuck out again, but this time, I was careful not to make the same mistake: I made sure the nurse didn't see me.

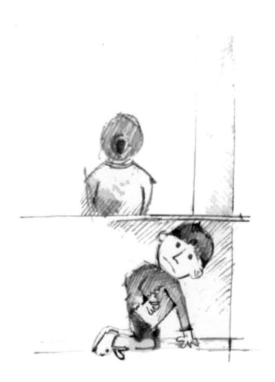

I passed in front of a room and saw the sunlight shining on many chairs. It was daytime, and the adults were asking me to sleep! There were many children sitting there; and each one had a bag, with a drug, hanging on a pole sitting next to them. There was a kind of hose, connected to the drug bag, carrying the drugs into their arm. I saw clear, red, and yellow drugs.

I talked to those kids and carefully took notes of everything they had learned from adults, and what they had heard among whispers. After that, I talked to adults. I approached them and told them it was useless to hide anything — as I had already found out a lot about cancer! They were kind, and then the nurse and other adults told me a lot of things. I'll tell you everything I know:

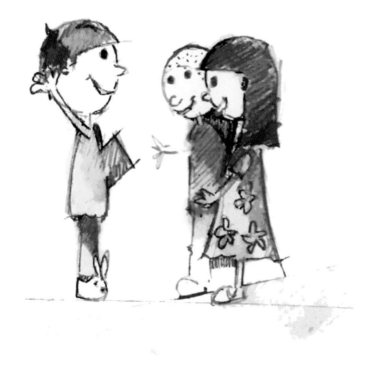

I discovered that cancer is a disease. I learned that we are all made of cells. One cell sits next to another, and together they form every part of our bodies. There are several types of cells; skin cells are different from heart cells, for example. All these cells grow, divide, and multiply: Several identical cells come from one cell.

I have found that cancer begins when a cell is transformed into a defective cell. This defective cell divides to create even more defected cells.

Sometimes, a defective cell can be born from a healthy cell and the body doesn't notice.

If the body doesn't notice the defect, the unhealthy cell can make other unhealthy cells, which can grow faster than healthy cells. They also need more nutrients than healthy cells. They press on parts of the body and cause damage to healthy cells.

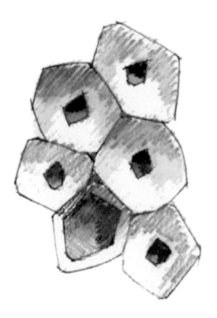

Because of that, the person may feel sick.

There are many types of cancer; and the type of a cancer depends on the body part where it was born. Some types cause more pain and disorder than others.

Some are easier to treat than others.

Some people take drugs by mouth.

Some people take drugs by the vein, which is like a little tube inside the arm. The vein carries the drug through the whole body.

Some drugs make a person bald, since the drug treats the whole body and can make hair fall out.

Those drugs that make hair fall out are not necessarily stronger than those that don't do it. There are many drugs that treat cancer. Different types of cancer are treated with different drugs. Each person is treated with the drug that works best to cure the type of cancer that they have.

The treatment is long, and it must be done exactly as the doctor orders.

Some people improve quickly; others, even with the drug, take a long time to get better.

All these people take other drugs too: to prevent pain and vomiting.

These people need to be treated with love, because they are sick.

These people can have a normal life. They can play, study, work, and be happy. They just cannot study and work when they are very ill.

When they are very ill, they recover in the hospital; but I saw a lot of people studying and working in the hospital too.

Sometimes people with cancer can run, play, and jump. Sometimes they may be very tired and ill. It depends on the type of illness and where they are in their treatment.

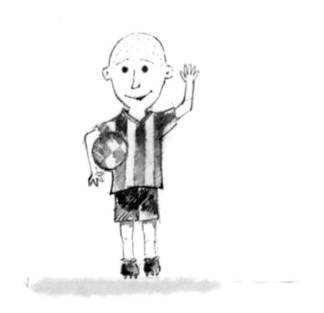

I also discovered the most important things: Cancer can be treated and cured. A person is beautiful even if they've lost their hair. I also learned how to live well and be happy: by not focusing on problems, dealing with the illness, and staying close to family and friends. And I discovered that adults just whisper because they don't know how to explain all of this to kids!

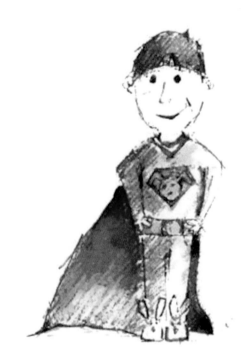

1st edition revised and updated - 3rd update
Print on demand